Smoothies For Weight Loss

Sip and Shed:
Delicious Smoothie Recipes
for
Effective Weight Loss

Lorraine Bond

TABLE OF CONTENTS

INTRODUCTION

In recent years, smoothies have gained immense popularity as a convenient and nutritious option for those seeking to manage their weight effectively. Packed with essential nutrients, vitamins, and minerals, smoothies offer a simple way to incorporate a variety of healthy ingredients into one delicious and easily digestible beverage. This introductory guide aims to provide an overview of how smoothies can be an integral part of a successful weight loss journey.

Smoothies are not only a delicious treat but can also serve as an effective tool for weight management. By carefully selecting the ingredients and portion sizes, smoothies can be tailored to support weight loss goals while providing the body with the necessary sustenance. Whether you are looking to shed a few pounds or maintain a healthy weight, incorporating smoothies into your diet can be a game-changer.

In this guide, we will explore the numerous benefits of smoothies for weight management, delve into the essential ingredients that make up a weight loss smoothie, and provide practical tips for incorporating smoothies into your daily routine. Additionally, we will introduce various types of smoothie recipes designed specifically for weight loss, including detoxifying green smoothies, protein-packed options for muscle maintenance, and low-calorie fruit-based recipes to satisfy sweet cravings without compromising on health.

Furthermore, we will discuss the concept of a 30-day smoothie challenge, offering a structured approach to kick-starting your weight loss journey and cultivating healthy habits. We will also highlight the role of nutrient-dense superfoods in smoothies and how they can contribute to overall health and weight control.

By the end of this guide, you will have a comprehensive understanding of how smoothies can be an integral part of your weight loss strategy and how to leverage their nutritional benefits to achieve your desired results. Whether you are new to the world of smoothies or looking to expand your repertoire, this guide will equip you with the knowledge and inspiration needed to embrace a healthy lifestyle through the power of weight loss smoothies.

Chapter 1: Essential Ingredients For Weight Loss Smoothies

When it comes to creating weight loss smoothies, incorporating essential ingredients that are nutrient-dense, low in calories, and high in fiber and protein is crucial. Here's a comprehensive list of essential ingredients for weight loss smoothies:

1. Leafy Greens:
   - Spinach, kale, Swiss chard, and collard greens are excellent choices. They are low in calories, high in fiber, and packed with vitamins, minerals, and antioxidants.

2. Fruits:
   - Berries (strawberries, blueberries, raspberries) are low in sugar and high in fiber and antioxidants.

- Apples and pears are also great options due to their high fiber content.

- Citrus fruits like oranges, lemons, and limes add a zesty flavor and are rich in vitamin C.

- Avocado provides healthy fats and a creamy texture without adding too much sugar.

3. Protein Sources:

- Greek yogurt: High in protein and probiotics, which can aid digestion and support a healthy gut.

- Nut butters (almond butter, peanut butter): Provide protein and healthy fats.

- Protein powder (whey, pea protein, hemp protein): Helps increase satiety and supports muscle recovery and growth.

4. Healthy Fats:
   -        Avocado: Rich   in
monounsaturated fats that promote
heart health and help keep you feeling
full.
   - Chia seeds, flaxseeds, hemp seeds:
Excellent sources of omega-3 fatty
acids and fiber.

5. Liquid Base:
   -      Unsweetened   almond   milk,
coconut milk, or oat milk: Low in
calories and can add creaminess to
the smoothie.
   - Coconut water: Provides hydration
and natural sweetness without added
sugars.

6. Fiber Boosters:
   - Flaxseeds, chia seeds, psyllium
husk: These can help promote
feelings of fullness and aid in
digestion.

7. Superfoods:
  - Matcha powder: Provides a natural energy boost and is rich in antioxidants.
  - Spirulina: A nutrient-dense algae that can support detoxification and provide essential nutrients.
  - Turmeric: Known for its anti-inflammatory properties.

8. Flavor Enhancers:
  - Fresh ginger: Adds a zingy flavor and may aid digestion.
  - Cinnamon: Adds warmth and sweetness without added sugar.

9. Sweeteners (optional):
  - Honey, agave nectar, or pitted dates can be used sparingly to sweeten the smoothie naturally.

10. Ice or Frozen Ingredients:

   - Adding ice or frozen fruits can create a thicker texture and a refreshing chill.

When creating weight loss smoothies, it's important to focus on portion control and balance. While these ingredients can support weight loss goals, it's essential to be mindful of overall calorie intake and ensure that the smoothie fits into a well-rounded, balanced diet. Additionally, consulting with a healthcare professional or nutritionist can provide personalized guidance based on individual health needs and goals.

Chapter 2: 30-day smoothie challenge for weight loss

A 30-day smoothie challenge is a commitment to drinking at least one smoothie a day for 30 days. The goal is to replace one meal or snack with a nutrient-dense smoothie and incorporate a variety of fruits, vegetables, protein, and healthy fats into your diet. This challenge is designed to jumpstart your weight loss by providing your body with a concentrated dose of essential vitamins and minerals.

Benefits of a 30-day smoothie challenge for weight loss:

1. Provides a concentrated dose of nutrients:
Smoothies are an excellent way to pack in a variety of nutrients into one meal. They are usually made with a

combination of fruits, vegetables, protein, and healthy fats, making them a complete and balanced meal. This ensures that your body is receiving all the necessary vitamins and minerals it needs to function properly, which can aid in weight loss.

2. Reduces cravings:
One of the biggest challenges when trying to lose weight is controlling cravings for unhealthy foods. By replacing one meal or snack with a smoothie, you are reducing the number of processed and unhealthy foods in your diet. The high fiber and protein content in smoothies can also help to keep you feeling full and satisfied, reducing cravings for unhealthy snacks and helping you stick to your weight loss goals.

3. Boosts metabolism:

Many ingredients commonly used in smoothies, such as leafy greens, berries, and protein, have been shown to boost metabolism. This means that your body will be able to burn calories more efficiently, aiding in weight loss. Smoothies are also easy to digest, allowing your body to absorb the nutrients quickly and provide you with sustained energy throughout the day.

4. Encourages healthy eating habits:
A 30-day smoothie challenge can help to kickstart healthier eating habits. By incorporating a variety of fruits and vegetables into your diet, you are training your taste buds to enjoy and crave healthier options. This can lead to sustainable weight loss and healthier eating choices in the long term.

How to do a 30-day smoothie challenge for weight loss:

1. Choose a high-quality blender:
Investing in a good blender is essential for a successful smoothie challenge. Look for a blender that is powerful enough to blend frozen fruits and vegetables and has multiple speed options to blend ingredients smoothly.

2. Choose your ingredients:
To make your smoothie nutrient-dense, choose a variety of fruits and vegetables such as berries, leafy greens, avocado, and bananas. Add in a source of protein, such as Greek yogurt, tofu, or protein powder, and a healthy fat like chia seeds, flaxseeds, or nut butter. You can also add in superfoods like spirulina, maca powder, or turmeric for extra health benefits.

3. Plan your smoothie recipes:

Having a variety of smoothie recipes planned out for the 30-day challenge can help to keep things interesting and prevent boredom. Search for recipes online or get creative and come up with your own recipe combinations using the ingredients you have chosen. Aim for a balanced mix of flavors and nutrients in each smoothie.

4. Replace one meal or snack with a smoothie:
To see maximum results, it's important to replace one meal or snack with a smoothie each day. Choose a time of day that works best for you and stick to it. This can be a breakfast smoothie to start your day off with a boost of energy, a mid-morning snack, or a post-workout meal.

5. Stay hydrated:

In addition to drinking your smoothies, it's essential to stay hydrated by drinking plenty of water throughout the day. This will help to flush out toxins, keep you feeling full, and aid in weight loss.

6. Listen to your body:
Listen to your body and make adjustments if needed. If you feel hungry, add more protein or healthy fats to your smoothies. If you feel like you need more variety, experiment with different ingredients and recipes. It's important to listen to your body's needs and make adjustments accordingly.

Tips for a successful 30-day smoothie challenge for weight loss:

1. Prep ahead: Save time and make your smoothie preparation easier by prepping ingredients ahead of time. Wash and chop fruits and vegetables, portion out protein and healthy fats, and freeze them in individual serving sizes.

2. Experiment with different ingredients: Don't be afraid to mix things up and try new ingredients in your smoothies. This will keep things interesting and ensure you are getting a variety of nutrients.

3. Make it a group challenge: Consider involving your friends or family members in the challenge to stay motivated and hold each other accountable.

4. Take progress pictures: Take photos of yourself at the beginning,

midpoint, and end of the challenge to track your progress and see the physical changes in your body.

5. Stay active: Pair your smoothie challenge with daily physical activity to maximize its effectiveness and achieve your weight loss goals.

Chapter 3: Green smoothie recipes for detox and weight loss

Green smoothies have become a popular choice for those looking to detox and lose weight. These nutrient-dense drinks are packed with vitamins, minerals, and antioxidants, and are a great way to start your day or include as a meal replacement. Here are 20 delicious green smoothie recipes that you can try at home for a refreshing and healthy boost.

1. Green Goddess Detox Smoothie
Ingredients:
- 1 cup spinach
- ½ cup kale
- ½ avocado
- 1 banana
- 1 cup almond milk

- 1 tsp ginger
- ½ tsp turmeric
- Juice of 1 lemon

Instructions:

1. Blend all ingredients until smooth and creamy.

2. Add a splash of water or more almond milk if needed to reach desired consistency.

3. Enjoy as a refreshing and detoxifying breakfast or snack.

2. Tropical Detox Smoothie

Ingredients:

- 1 cup spinach
- ½ cup pineapple
- ½ cup mango
- 1 banana
- 1 cup coconut water
- 1 tbsp chia seeds

Instructions:

1. Blend all ingredients until smooth and creamy.

2. If the smoothie is too thick, add more coconut water to thin it out.

3. Decorate with a slice of pineapple or mango for an extra tropical touch.

3. Green Detox Power Smoothie
Ingredients:
- 1 cup kale
- 1 cup spinach
- ½ cup cucumber
- ½ avocado
- 1 celery stalk
- 1 apple
- 1 tbsp flax seeds
- 1 cup water

Instructions:
1. Blend all ingredients until smooth and creamy.

2. Add more water if needed for desired consistency.

3. This highly nutritious and filling smoothie is perfect for a meal replacement during a detox.

4. Berry Blast Detox Smoothie
Ingredients:
- ½ cup spinach
- ½ cup kale
- ½ cup strawberries
- ½ cup blueberries
- 1 banana
- 1 cup almond milk
- 1 tbsp almond butter

Instructions:
1. Blend all ingredients until smooth and creamy.
2. For a thicker smoothie, use frozen berries and less almond milk.
3. Enjoy this antioxidant-rich smoothie as a snack or a refreshing post-workout drink.

5. Green Tea Detox Smoothie
Ingredients:
- 1 cup spinach
- ½ cup cucumber
- 1 green apple
- 1 tsp matcha green tea powder
- 1 cup green tea, brewed and chilled
- 1 tbsp honey

Instructions:
1. Blend all ingredients until smooth and creamy.
2. Serve over ice for a refreshing and energizing detox drink.

6. Cucumber and Mint Detox Smoothie
Ingredients:
- 1 cup spinach
- ½ cup cucumber
- ½ avocado
- 1 banana
- 1 cup coconut water
- 1 tbsp mint leaves

- Juice of 1 lime

Instructions:
1. Blend all ingredients until smooth and creamy.
2. Add more coconut water for a thinner consistency.
3. The refreshing combination of cucumber and mint makes this smoothie perfect for a hot summer day.

7. Pineapple and Ginger Detox Smoothie
Ingredients:
- 1 cup spinach
- ½ cup pineapple
- ½ avocado
- 1 banana
- 1 tbsp fresh ginger, grated
- 1 cup coconut water

Instructions:

1. Blend all ingredients until smooth and creamy.

2. If the smoothie is too thick, add more coconut water to thin it out.

3. The anti-inflammatory properties of ginger make this smoothie great for reducing bloating and aiding digestion.

8. Kale and Kiwi Detox Smoothie

Ingredients:

- 1 cup kale
- 1 kiwi, peeled
- 1 banana
- 1 cup almond milk
- 1 tbsp hemp seeds

Instructions:

1. Blend all ingredients until smooth and creamy.

2. Add more almond milk for a thinner consistency.

3. This vitamin-C rich smoothie is perfect for boosting your immune system and fighting off toxins.

9. Avocado and Spirulina Detox Smoothie
Ingredients:
- 1 cup spinach
- ½ avocado
- 1 banana
- 1 tsp spirulina powder
- 1 cup almond milk
- 1 tbsp honey

Instructions:
1. Blend all ingredients until smooth and creamy.
2. Add more almond milk if needed for desired consistency.
3. This smoothie is loaded with healthy fats and detoxifying properties from the avocado and spirulina.

10. Carrot and Orange Detox Smoothie

Ingredients:

- 1 cup spinach
- 1 carrot, peeled and chopped
- 1 orange, peeled and chopped
- 1 banana
- 1 cup water
- 1 tbsp ginger, grated

Instructions:

1. Blend all ingredients until smooth and creamy.
2. Add more water for a thinner consistency.
3. This vibrant smoothie is rich in vitamin A, C, and antioxidants, making it great for clear skin and detoxifying the body.

11. Blueberry and Beet Detox Smoothie

Ingredients:

- ½ cup spinach
- ½ cup beet, cooked and chopped
- ½ cup blueberries
- 1 banana
- 1 cup almond milk
- 1 tbsp chia seeds

Instructions:

1. Blend all ingredients until smooth and creamy.
2. For a thicker smoothie, use frozen blueberries and less almond milk.
3. The detoxifying properties of beets make this smoothie perfect for a post-workout recovery drink.

12. Melon and Mint Detox Smoothie

Ingredients:

- 1 cup spinach
- 1 cup honeydew melon, diced

- 1 banana
- 1 tbsp fresh mint leaves
- 1 cup coconut water
- Juice of 1 lime

Instructions:
1. Blend all ingredients until smooth and creamy.
2. Add more coconut water if needed for desired consistency.
3. The refreshing combination of melon and mint make this smoothie perfect for a summer detox drink.

13. Spinach and Pear Detox Smoothie
Ingredients:
- 1 cup spinach
- 1 pear, peeled and chopped
- 1 banana
- 1 cup almond milk
- 1 tbsp almond butter

Instructions:
1. Blend all ingredients until smooth and creamy.
2. Add more almond milk for a thinner consistency.
3. The healthy combination of pear and spinach makes this smoothie a great choice for a meal replacement during a detox.

14. Papaya and Coconut Detox Smoothie
Ingredients:
- 1 cup spinach
- ½ cup papaya, diced
- ½ avocado
- 1 banana
- 1 cup coconut milk
- 1 tbsp shredded coconut

Instructions:
1. Blend all ingredients until smooth and creamy.

2. Add more coconut milk for a thinner consistency.

3. This tropical smoothie is rich in fibers and healthy fats, making it great for improving digestion and supporting weight loss.

15. Matcha and Mango Detox Smoothie

Ingredients:
- 1 cup spinach
- 1 cup frozen mango
- 1 banana
- 1 tsp matcha green tea powder
- 1 cup almond milk

Instructions:
1. Blend all ingredients until smooth and creamy.

2. For a thicker smoothie, use frozen mango and less almond milk.

3. The antioxidant-rich matcha powder adds a boost of energy and

detoxifying properties to this delicious smoothie.

16. Chocolate Avocado Detox Smoothie

Ingredients:
- 1 cup spinach
- ½ avocado
- 1 banana
- 1 tbsp cacao powder
- 1 cup almond milk
- 1 tbsp honey

Instructions:
1. Blend all ingredients until smooth and creamy.
2. Add more almond milk for a thinner consistency.
3. The healthy fats from avocado and the antioxidant properties of cacao make this smoothie a delicious and nutritious choice for a detox.

17. Apple and Broccoli Detox Smoothie

Ingredients:

- 1 cup broccoli florets
- ½ green apple, chopped
- 1 banana
- 1 cup almond milk
- 1 tbsp honey

Instructions:

1. Blend all ingredients until smooth and creamy.
2. Add more almond milk if needed for desired consistency.
3. This smoothie is rich in fiber and nutrients from the combination of broccoli and apple, making it great for digestion and detoxification.

18. Grapefruit and Ginger Detox Smoothie

Ingredients:

- 1 cup spinach
- ½ grapefruit, peeled and chopped

- ½ avocado
- 1 banana
- 1 tsp fresh ginger, grated
- 1 cup coconut water

Instructions:

1. Blend all ingredients until smooth and creamy.

2. Add more coconut water for a thinner consistency.

3. The detoxifying properties of grapefruit and ginger make this smoothie perfect for a refreshing breakfast or snack.

19. Oat and Banana Detox Smoothie

Ingredients:

- 1 cup spinach
- ½ cup rolled oats
- 1 banana
- 1 tbsp almond butter
- 1 cup almond milk
- 1 tsp cinnamon

Instructions:

1. Blend all ingredients until smooth and creamy.

2. For a thicker smoothie, use less almond milk.

3. The combination of fiber from oats and potassium from banana make this smoothie great for a healthy digestion and weight loss.

20. Spinach and Pineapple Detox Smoothie

Ingredients:

- 1 cup spinach
- ½ cup pineapple
- 1 banana
- 1 cup coconut water
- Juice of 1 lemon
- 1 tbsp coconut oil

Instructions:

1. Blend all ingredients until smooth and creamy.

2. Add more coconut water for a thinner consistency.

3. The addition of coconut oil adds healthy fats and aids in the detoxification process,

Chapter 4: Protein-packed smoothies for lean muscle and fat loss

1. Banana Almond Protein Shake

Ingredients:
- 1 banana
- ½ cup almond milk
- ½ cup Greek yogurt
- 1 scoop vanilla protein powder
- 1 tbsp almond butter

Instructions:
1. In a blender, add the banana, almond milk, Greek yogurt, protein powder, and almond butter.
2. Blend until smooth and creamy.
3. Pour into a glass and enjoy!

2. Strawberry Kiwi Protein Smoothie

Ingredients:
- ½ cup frozen strawberries
- ½ cup frozen kiwi
- 1 cup spinach
- ½ cup unsweetened almond milk
- 1 scoop vanilla protein powder

Instructions:
1. In a blender, add the frozen strawberries, frozen kiwi, spinach, almond milk, and protein powder.
2. Blend until smooth.
3. Pour into a glass and enjoy!

3. Chocolate Peanut Butter Protein Shake

Ingredients:
- 1 cup unsweetened almond milk
- 1 scoop chocolate protein powder
- 1 banana
- 1 tbsp peanut butter
- Handful of ice cubes

Instructions:

1. In a blender, add the almond milk, protein powder, banana, peanut butter, and ice cubes.
2. Blend until smooth and creamy.
3. Pour into a glass and enjoy!

4. Green Machine Protein Smoothie
Ingredients:
- 1 cup unsweetened coconut water
- 1 scoop vanilla protein powder
- 1 cup kale
- ½ cup frozen mango
- ½ avocado

Instructions:
1. In a blender, add the coconut water, protein powder, kale, frozen mango, and avocado.
2. Blend until smooth.
3. Pour into a glass and enjoy!

5. Blueberry Oatmeal Protein Shake

Ingredients:
- 1 cup unsweetened almond milk
- 1 scoop vanilla protein powder
- ½ cup frozen blueberries
- ¼ cup rolled oats
- Handful of ice cubes

Instructions:
1. In a blender, add the almond milk, protein powder, frozen blueberries, rolled oats, and ice cubes.
2. Blend until smooth and creamy.
3. Pour into a glass and enjoy!

6. Mango Coconut Protein Smoothie

Ingredients:
- 1 cup unsweetened coconut milk
- 1 scoop vanilla protein powder
- 1 cup frozen mango
- ½ cup Greek yogurt
- 1 tbsp shredded coconut

Instructions:

1. In a blender, add the coconut milk, protein powder, frozen mango, Greek yogurt, and shredded coconut.
2. Blend until smooth.
3. Pour into a glass and enjoy!

7. Chocolate Cherry Protein Shake

Ingredients:

- 1 cup unsweetened almond milk
- 1 scoop chocolate protein powder
- 1 cup frozen cherries
- ½ banana
- Handful of spinach

Instructions:

1. In a blender, add the almond milk, protein powder, frozen cherries, banana, and spinach.
2. Blend until smooth and creamy.
3. Pour into a glass and enjoy!

8. Peanut Butter Banana Protein Smoothie
Ingredients:
- 1 cup unsweetened almond milk
- 1 scoop vanilla protein powder
- 1 banana
- 1 tbsp peanut butter
- Handful of spinach

Instructions:
1. In a blender, add the almond milk, protein powder, banana, peanut butter, and spinach.
2. Blend until smooth.
3. Pour into a glass and enjoy!

9. Raspberry Chia Seed Protein Shake
Ingredients:
- ½ cup unsweetened almond milk
- 1 scoop vanilla protein powder
- 1 cup raspberries
- 1 tbsp chia seeds
- Handful of ice cubes

Instructions:

1. In a blender, add the almond milk, protein powder, raspberries, chia seeds, and ice cubes.
2. Blend until smooth and creamy.
3. Pour into a glass and enjoy!

10. Avocado Protein Smoothie

Ingredients:

- 1 cup unsweetened almond milk
- 1 scoop vanilla protein powder
- ½ avocado
- ½ cup Greek yogurt
- 1 tsp honey

Instructions:

1. In a blender, add the almond milk, protein powder, avocado, Greek yogurt, and honey.
2. Blend until smooth.
3. Pour into a glass and enjoy!

11. Orange Creamsicle Protein Shake

Ingredients:
- 1 cup unsweetened almond milk
- 1 scoop vanilla protein powder
- 1 orange, peeled
- ½ banana
- Handful of ice cubes

Instructions:
1. In a blender, add the almond milk, protein powder, orange, banana, and ice cubes.
2. Blend until smooth and creamy.
3. Pour into a glass and enjoy!

12. Berry Blast Protein Smoothie

Ingredients:
- 1 cup unsweetened coconut water
- 1 scoop vanilla protein powder
- ½ cup frozen mixed berries
- ½ cup frozen pineapple
- Handful of spinach

Instructions:

1. In a blender, add the coconut water, protein powder, frozen mixed berries, frozen pineapple, and spinach.
2. Blend until smooth.
3. Pour into a glass and enjoy!

13. Chocolate Banana Nut Protein Shake

Ingredients:
- 1 cup unsweetened almond milk
- 1 scoop chocolate protein powder
- 1 banana
- 1 tbsp almond butter
- 1 tbsp chopped walnuts

Instructions:

1. In a blender, add the almond milk, protein powder, banana, almond butter, and chopped walnuts.
2. Blend until smooth and creamy.
3. Pour into a glass and enjoy!

14. Peach Oatmeal Protein Smoothie

Ingredients:

- 1 cup unsweetened almond milk
- 1 scoop vanilla protein powder
- 1 cup frozen peaches
- ¼ cup rolled oats
- Handful of ice cubes

Instructions:

1. In a blender, add the almond milk, protein powder, frozen peaches, rolled oats, and ice cubes.
2. Blend until smooth.
3. Pour into a glass and enjoy!

15. Tropical Green Protein Shake

Ingredients:

- 1 cup unsweetened coconut milk
- 1 scoop vanilla protein powder
- ½ cup frozen pineapple
- ½ cup frozen mango

- Handful of spinach

Instructions:
1. In a blender, add the coconut milk, protein powder, frozen pineapple, frozen mango, and spinach.
2. Blend until smooth and creamy.
3. Pour into a glass and enjoy!

16. Vanilla Almond Protein Smoothie
Ingredients:
- 1 cup unsweetened almond milk
- 1 scoop vanilla protein powder
- 1 banana
- 1 tbsp almond butter
- 1 tsp honey

Instructions:
1. In a blender, add the almond milk, protein powder, banana, almond butter, and honey.
2. Blend until smooth.
3. Pour into a glass and enjoy!

17. Blueberry Banana Protein Shake

Ingredients:
- 1 cup unsweetened almond milk
- 1 scoop vanilla protein powder
- ½ cup frozen blueberries
- ½ banana
- Handful of spinach

Instructions:
1. In a blender, add the almond milk, protein powder, frozen blueberries, banana, and spinach.
2. Blend until smooth and creamy.
3. Pour into a glass and enjoy!

18. PB&J Protein Smoothie

Ingredients:
- 1 cup unsweetened almond milk
- 1 scoop vanilla protein powder
- ½ cup frozen strawberries
- 1 tbsp peanut butter
- 1 tbsp chia seeds

Instructions:

1. In a blender, add the almond milk, protein powder, frozen strawberries, peanut butter, and chia seeds.
2. Blend until smooth.
3. Pour into a glass and enjoy!

19. Chocolate Cherry Coconut Protein Shake

Ingredients:

- 1 cup unsweetened coconut water
- 1 scoop chocolate protein powder
- 1 cup frozen cherries
- 1 tbsp shredded coconut
- Handful of ice cubes

Instructions:

1. In a blender, add the coconut water, protein powder, frozen cherries, shredded coconut, and ice cubes.
2. Blend until smooth and creamy.
3. Pour into a glass and enjoy!

20. Strawberry Banana Chia Protein Smoothie

Ingredients:
- 1 cup unsweetened almond milk
- 1 scoop vanilla protein powder
- 1 banana
- 1 cup frozen strawberries
- 1 tbsp chia seeds

Instructions:

1. In a blender, add the almond milk, protein powder, banana, frozen strawberries, and chia seeds.
2. Blend until smooth.
3. Pour into a glass and enjoy!

Chapter 5: Low-calorie fruit smoothies for satisfying sweet cravings

1. Strawberry Banana Smoothie
Ingredients:
- 1 cup frozen strawberries
- 1 frozen banana
- 1 cup unsweetened almond milk
- 1 tbsp chia seeds
- 1 tbsp honey
- 1 tsp vanilla extract

Instructions:
1. Add all ingredients to a blender.
2. Blend until smooth and creamy.
3. Serve and enjoy!

2. Peach Mango Smoothie
Ingredients:
- 1 cup frozen peaches
- 1 cup frozen mango
- 1 cup unsweetened coconut water
- ½ cup Greek yogurt

- 1 tbsp honey
- Juice of ½ lime

Instructions:
1. Add all ingredients to a blender.
2. Blend until smooth and creamy.
3. Serve and enjoy!

3. Blueberry Spinach Smoothie
Ingredients:
- 1 cup frozen blueberries
- 1 cup fresh spinach
- 1 cup unsweetened almond milk
- 1 tbsp flaxseed meal
- 1 tbsp honey
- ½ tsp cinnamon

Instructions:
1. Add all ingredients to a blender.
2. Blend until smooth and creamy.
3. Serve and enjoy!

4. Peach Raspberry Smoothie
Ingredients:

- 1 cup frozen peaches
- 1 cup frozen raspberries
- 1 cup unsweetened coconut water
- ¼ cup plain Greek yogurt
- 1 tbsp maple syrup
- Ice (optional)

Instructions:
1. Add all ingredients to a blender.
2. Blend until smooth and creamy.
3. If desired, add ice for a thicker consistency.
4. Serve and enjoy!

5. Green Apple Kale Smoothie
Ingredients:
- 1 cup chopped green apple
- 1 cup fresh kale
- 1 cup unsweetened almond milk
- 1 tbsp almond butter
- 1 tsp honey
- ½ tsp ground ginger

Instructions:
1. Add all ingredients to a blender.

2. Blend until smooth and creamy.

3. Serve and enjoy!

6. Strawberry Pineapple Smoothie

Ingredients:
- 1 cup frozen strawberries
- 1 cup frozen pineapple
- 1 cup unsweetened coconut water
- ½ cup plain Greek yogurt
- 1 tbsp honey
- Juice of ½ lemon

Instructions:
1. Add all ingredients to a blender.
2. Blend until smooth and creamy.
3. Serve and enjoy!

7. Mango Avocado Smoothie
Ingredients:
- 1 cup frozen mango
- ½ avocado
- 1 cup unsweetened almond milk
- 1 tbsp honey

- ½ tsp turmeric
- 1 tsp fresh ginger

Instructions:
1. Add all ingredients to a blender.
2. Blend until smooth and creamy.
3. Serve and enjoy!

8. Cherry Almond Smoothie
Ingredients:
- 1 cup frozen cherries
- 1 banana
- 1 cup unsweetened almond milk
- 1 tbsp almond butter
- 1 tbsp honey
- ½ tsp almond extract

Instructions:
1. Add all ingredients to a blender.
2. Blend until smooth and creamy.
3. Serve and enjoy!

9. Raspberry Coconut Smoothie
Ingredients:

- 1 cup frozen raspberries
- 1 frozen banana
- 1 cup unsweetened coconut milk
- ¼ cup plain Greek yogurt
- 1 tbsp honey
- ½ tsp vanilla extract

Instructions:
1. Add all ingredients to a blender.
2. Blend until smooth and creamy.
3. Serve and enjoy!

10. Peach Pear Smoothie
Ingredients:
- 1 cup frozen peaches
- 1 pear
- 1 cup unsweetened almond milk
- 1 tbsp flaxseed meal
- 1 tbsp honey
- ½ tsp cinnamon

Instructions:
1. Add all ingredients to a blender.

2. Blend until smooth and creamy.
3. Serve and enjoy!

11. Triple Berry Smoothie
Ingredients:
- 1 cup frozen mixed berries
- 1 frozen banana
- 1 cup unsweetened almond milk
- ½ cup plain Greek yogurt
- 1 tbsp honey
- Juice of ½ lime

Instructions:
1. Add all ingredients to a blender.
2. Blend until smooth and creamy.
3. Serve and enjoy!

12. Pineapple Coconut Smoothie
Ingredients:
- 1 cup frozen pineapple
- ½ cup frozen mango
- 1 cup unsweetened coconut milk
- 1 tbsp chia seeds
- 1 tbsp honey

- ½ tsp coconut extract

Instructions:
1. Add all ingredients to a blender.
2. Blend until smooth and creamy.
3. Serve and enjoy!

13. Orange Carrot Smoothie
Ingredients:
- 1 large orange
- 1 large carrot, peeled and chopped
- 1 cup unsweetened almond milk
- 1 tbsp honey
- ½ tsp ground turmeric
- 1 tsp fresh ginger

Instructions:
1. Add all ingredients to a blender.
2. Blend until smooth and creamy.
3. Serve and enjoy!

14. Banana Peach Green Smoothie
Ingredients:

- 1 frozen banana
- 1 cup frozen peaches
- 1 cup fresh baby spinach
- 1 cup unsweetened almond milk
- 1 tbsp almond butter
- 1 tbsp honey

Instructions:
1. Add all ingredients to a blender.
2. Blend until smooth and creamy.
3. Serve and enjoy!

15. Mixed Berry Oat Smoothie
Ingredients:
- 1 cup frozen mixed berries
- ½ cup rolled oats
- 1 cup unsweetened almond milk
- 1 tbsp honey
- ½ tsp vanilla extract

Instructions:
1. Add all ingredients to a blender.
2. Blend until smooth and creamy.

3. Serve and enjoy!

16. Cherry Vanilla Smoothie
Ingredients:
- 1 cup frozen cherries
- 1 frozen banana
- 1 cup unsweetened almond milk
- ½ cup plain Greek yogurt
- 1 tbsp honey
- ½ tsp vanilla extract

Instructions:
1. Add all ingredients to a blender.
2. Blend until smooth and creamy.
3. Serve and enjoy!

17. Pineapple Mango Coconut Smoothie
Ingredients:
- 1 cup frozen pineapple
- 1 cup frozen mango
- 1 cup unsweetened coconut milk
- 1 tbsp honey
- 1 tbsp chia seeds

- ½ tsp coconut extract

Instructions:
1. Add all ingredients to a blender.
2. Blend until smooth and creamy.
3. Serve and enjoy!

18. Blueberry Almond Smoothie
Ingredients:
- 1 cup frozen blueberries
- ½ frozen banana
- 1 cup unsweetened almond milk
- 1 tbsp almond butter
- 1 tbsp honey
- 1 tsp fresh lemon juice

Instructions:
1. Add all ingredients to a blender.
2. Blend until smooth and creamy.
3. Serve and enjoy!

19. Kiwi Strawberry Smoothie
Ingredients:
- 2 kiwi, peeled and diced

- 1 cup frozen strawberries
- 1 cup unsweetened almond milk
- 1 tbsp honey
- ½ tsp ginger
- 1 tsp fresh lime juice

Instructions:
1. Add all ingredients to a blender.
2. Blend until smooth and creamy.
3. Serve and enjoy!

20. Turmeric Mango Smoothie

Ingredients:
- 1 cup frozen mango
- 1 cup unsweetened coconut milk
- 1 tbsp honey
- 1 tbsp chia seeds
- 1 tsp ground turmeric
- ½ tsp fresh ginger

Instructions:
1. Add all ingredients to a blender.
2. Blend until smooth and creamy.

3. Serve and enjoy!

Chapter 6: Nutrient-dense super food smoothies for overall health and weight control

1. Green Goddess Smoothie
Ingredients:
- 1 cup spinach
- ½ avocado
- 1 banana
- 1 tbsp chia seeds
- 1 tbsp hemp seeds
- 1 cup almond milk
- ½ tsp grated ginger
- 1 tsp honey (optional)

Instructions:
1. In a blender, add spinach, avocado, banana, chia seeds, hemp seeds, almond milk, ginger, and honey if desired.
2. Blend until smooth and creamy.

3. Serve and enjoy the nutrient-packed green goddess smoothie.

2. Berry Blast Smoothie
Ingredients:
- 1 cup mixed berries (strawberries, blueberries, raspberries)
- 1 banana
- 1 tbsp almond butter
- 1 tbsp flax seeds
- 1 cup coconut water
- ½ tsp cinnamon
- 1 tsp maple syrup (optional)

Instructions:
1. Put mixed berries, banana, almond butter, flax seeds, coconut water, cinnamon, and maple syrup if desired into a blender.
2. Blend until smooth and creamy.
3. Pour into a glass and enjoy this tasty and nutrient-rich berry blast smoothie.

3. Tropical Paradise Smoothie
Ingredients:
- 1 cup pineapple chunks
- 1 banana
- 1 cup coconut milk
- 1 tbsp shredded coconut
- 1 tbsp maca powder
- 1 tsp honey (optional)

Instructions:
1. Add pineapple chunks, banana, coconut milk, shredded coconut, maca powder, and honey if desired into a blender.
2. Blend until smooth and creamy.
3. Pour into a glass and enjoy the tropical flavors and health benefits of this smoothie.

4. Chocolate Banana Protein Smoothie
Ingredients:
- 1 cup almond milk
- 1 scoop chocolate protein powder

- 1 banana
- 1 tbsp peanut butter
- 1 tbsp cacao powder
- ½ tsp vanilla extract
- Ice cubes (optional)

Instructions:

1. In a blender, add almond milk, chocolate protein powder, banana, peanut butter, cacao powder, vanilla extract, and ice cubes if desired.
2. Blend until smooth and creamy.
3. Pour into a glass and enjoy this protein-packed and delicious smoothie.

5. Kale and Mango Power Smoothie

Ingredients:
- 1 cup kale
- 1 mango, diced
- ½ cup Greek yogurt

- 1 tbsp honey
- 1 tbsp almond butter
- 1 cup unsweetened almond milk
- ½ tsp turmeric
- ½ tsp grated ginger

Instructions:
1. Combine kale, mango, Greek yogurt, honey, almond butter, almond milk, turmeric, and ginger in a blender.
2. Blend until smooth and creamy.
3. Pour into a glass and enjoy this nutrient-dense and energizing smoothie.

6. Blueberry Oatmeal Smoothie
Ingredients:
- 1 cup blueberries
- ½ cup rolled oats
- 1 banana
- 1 cup unsweetened almond milk

- 1 tbsp honey
- 1 tsp cinnamon
- Ice cubes (optional)

Instructions:
1. Put blueberries, rolled oats, banana, almond milk, honey, cinnamon, and ice cubes if desired into a blender.
2. Blend until smooth and creamy.
3. Pour into a glass and enjoy this fiber-rich and delicious smoothie.

7. Creamy Carrot Cake Smoothie
Ingredients:
- 1 cup carrots, chopped
- 1 banana
- 1 cup unsweetened almond milk
- 1 tbsp almond butter
- 1 tbsp chia seeds
- 1 tsp maple syrup
- ½ tsp cinnamon
- ¼ tsp nutmeg

Instructions:

1. Add carrots, banana, almond milk, almond butter, chia seeds, maple syrup, cinnamon, and nutmeg into a blender.

2. Blend until smooth and creamy.

3. Pour into a glass and enjoy this tasty and nutrient-rich smoothie.

8. Superfood Green Smoothie

Ingredients:

- 1 cup spinach
- ½ cup kale
- ½ avocado
- ½ cup pineapple chunks
- 1 apple, chopped
- 1 tbsp chia seeds
- 1 cup coconut water
- ¼ tsp spirulina powder
- ½ tsp lemon juice

Instructions:

1. Combine spinach, kale, avocado, pineapple chunks, apple, chia seeds,

coconut water, spirulina powder, and lemon juice in a blender.

2. Blend until smooth and creamy.

3. Pour into a glass and enjoy this antioxidant-rich and detoxifying smoothie.

9. Vanilla Matcha Smoothie

Ingredients:
- 1 cup almond milk
- 1 banana
- 1 tbsp almond butter
- 1 tsp matcha powder
- ½ tsp vanilla extract
- 1 tsp honey (optional)

Instructions:

1. In a blender, add almond milk, banana, almond butter, matcha powder, vanilla extract, and honey if desired.

2. Blend until smooth and creamy.

3. Pour into a glass and enjoy this energizing and metabolism-boosting smoothie.

10. Pomegranate Ginger Smoothie

Ingredients:
- 1 cup pomegranate seeds
- 1 banana
- ½ inch fresh ginger, grated
- 1 tbsp hemp seeds
- 1 cup coconut water
- 1 tsp honey (optional)

Instructions:
1. Add pomegranate seeds, banana, fresh ginger, hemp seeds, coconut water, and honey if desired in a blender.
2. Blend until smooth and creamy.
3. Pour into a glass and enjoy this immune-boosting and anti-inflammatory smoothie.

11. Golden Turmeric Smoothie

Ingredients:

- 1 cup mango chunks
- 1 banana
- 1 tsp turmeric powder
- 1 tsp ginger powder
- ½ tsp cinnamon
- 1 cup coconut milk
- 1 tsp honey (optional)

Instructions:

1. Put mango chunks, banana, turmeric powder, ginger powder, cinnamon, coconut milk, and honey if desired into a blender.

2. Blend until smooth and creamy.

3. Pour into a glass and enjoy the anti-inflammatory and immune-boosting benefits of this golden turmeric smoothie.

12. Cucumber and Mint Smoothie

Ingredients:

- 1 cucumber
- 1 cup spinach
- ¼ cup fresh mint leaves
- ½ avocado
- 1 tbsp flax seeds
- 1 cup coconut water
- 1 tsp honey (optional)

Instructions:

1. Combine cucumber, spinach, mint leaves, avocado, flax seeds, coconut water, and honey if desired in a blender.

2. Blend until smooth and creamy.

3. Pour into a glass and enjoy this refreshing and nutrient-packed smoothie.

13. Peach and Ginger Smoothie

Ingredients:

- 1 cup frozen peaches
- ½ inch fresh ginger, grated
- 1 banana
- 1 tbsp almond butter

- 1 cup almond milk
- 1 tsp honey (optional)

Instructions:

1. In a blender, add frozen peaches, fresh ginger, banana, almond butter, almond milk, and honey if desired.
2. Blend until smooth and creamy.
3. Pour into a glass and enjoy the sweet and spicy flavors of this peach and ginger smoothie.

14. Chocolate Cherry Smoothie
Ingredients:

- 1 cup frozen cherries
- 1 banana
- 1 tbsp cacao powder
- ½ cup Greek yogurt
- 1 cup unsweetened almond milk
- 1 tsp honey (optional)

Instructions:

1. Combine frozen cherries, banana, cacao powder, Greek yogurt, almond milk, and honey if desired in a blender.

2. Blend until smooth and creamy.

3. Pour into a glass and enjoy this indulgent and protein-rich smoothie.

15. Coconut Berry Smoothie

Ingredients:

- 1 cup mixed berries (strawberries, blueberries, raspberries)
- ½ cup frozen cauliflower
- 1 banana
- 1 tbsp coconut oil
- 1 cup coconut water
- 1 tsp honey (optional)

Instructions:

1. Put mixed berries, frozen cauliflower, banana, coconut oil, coconut water, and honey if desired into a blender.

2. Blend until smooth and creamy.

3. Pour into a glass and enjoy this creamy and nutrient-dense smoothie.

16. Mango and Turmeric Smoothie

Ingredients:
- 1 cup mango chunks
- 1 banana
- ½ tsp turmeric powder
- 1 tsp grated ginger
- ½ cup Greek yogurt
- 1 cup unsweetened almond milk
- 1 tsp honey (optional)

Instructions:
1. Add mango chunks, banana, turmeric powder, grated ginger, Greek yogurt, almond milk, and honey if desired into a blender.
2. Blend until smooth and creamy.
3. Pour into a glass and enjoy this anti-inflammatory and digestive health-promoting smoothie.

17. Peanut Butter Banana Smoothie

Ingredients:

- 1 banana
- 1 tbsp peanut butter
- 1 cup unsweetened almond milk
- 1 scoop vanilla protein powder
- 1 tsp honey (optional)
- Ice cubes (optional)

Instructions:

1. In a blender, add banana, peanut butter, almond milk, protein powder, honey if desired, and ice cubes if desired.

2. Blend until smooth and creamy.

3. Pour into a glass and enjoy this protein-packed and satisfying smoothie.

18. Strawberry Coconut Chia Smoothie

Ingredients:

- 1 cup frozen strawberries
- ½ cup coconut milk
- 1 tbsp chia seeds
- 1 banana
- 1 tsp honey (optional)

Instructions:

1. Combine frozen strawberries, coconut milk, chia seeds, banana, and honey if desired in a blender.
2. Blend until smooth and creamy.
3. Pour into a glass and enjoy this creamy and antioxidant-rich smoothie.

19. Spinach and Pineapple Detox Smoothie

Ingredients:

- 1 cup spinach
- ½ cup pineapple chunks
- 1 green apple

- 1 tbsp lemon juice
- 1 tsp grated ginger
- ½ tsp spirulina powder
- 1 cup coconut water
- 1 tsp honey (optional)

Instructions:

1. In a blender, add spinach, pineapple chunks, green apple, lemon juice, grated ginger, spirulina powder, coconut water, and honey if desired.

2. Blend until smooth and creamy.

3. Pour into a glass and enjoy this detoxifying and refreshing smoothie.

20. Pumpkin Spice Smoothie
Ingredients:
- 1 cup pumpkin puree
- 1 banana
- 1 tsp pumpkin pie spice
- ½ tsp vanilla extract
- 1 cup unsweetened almond milk
- 1 tsp maple syrup (optional)

Instructions:

1. Combine pumpkin puree, banana, pumpkin pie spice, vanilla extract, almond milk, and maple syrup if desired in a blender.
2. Blend until smooth and creamy.
3. Pour into a glass and savor the flavors of fall with this pumpkin spice smoothie.

Chapter 7: Tips for incorporating smoothies into a weight loss diet

Smoothies have gained immense popularity in recent years as a convenient and delicious way to get a quick dose of nutrition. However, did you know that smoothies can also be a powerful tool for weight loss? Yes, you read it right! With the right combination of ingredients, smoothies can not only help you shed those stubborn extra pounds but also provide you with essential nutrients that your body needs. Here are some tips for incorporating smoothies into your weight loss diet:

1. Choose the Right Base

The base of your smoothie is the key to its texture and consistency. To keep your smoothie low in calories and fat, opt for a low-fat or plant-based milk like almond milk, coconut milk, or oat milk. You can also use water or green tea as the base for your smoothie. Avoid using high-fat dairy products like full-fat milk or yogurt, as they can add unnecessary calories to your smoothie.

2. Load Up on Low-Calorie Vegetables

Vegetables are an excellent addition to any smoothie, not only for their nutritional value but also because they are low in calories. Some good options to add to your smoothie include spinach, kale, lettuce, cucumber, and celery. These vegetables are rich in fiber and water, which can help you stay full for longer and prevent overeating.

3. Don't Forget the Protein

Protein is an essential nutrient for weight loss as it helps in building and repairing muscles, which in turn, boosts metabolism. To make your smoothie more filling and satisfying, add a scoop of protein powder, Greek yogurt, or tofu. You can also add nuts and seeds like almonds, chia seeds, or hemp seeds, which are not only a good source of protein but also provide healthy fats and fiber.

4. Add Some Healthy Fats

Healthy fats are crucial for the smooth functioning of our body and contribute to weight loss as well. Adding a small amount of avocado, coconut oil, or nut butter to your smoothie can provide healthy fats and make your smoothie more satisfying. However, remember to keep the serving size in check as these ingredients are high in calories.

5. Skip the Artificial Sweeteners

While it may be tempting to add some artificial sweeteners to your smoothie, it is best to avoid them. Artificial sweeteners have zero calories but can have a negative impact on your weight loss goals. They can trigger sugar cravings, causing you to consume more calories throughout the day. Instead, opt for natural sweeteners like honey, dates, or mashed banana to add some sweetness to your smoothie.

6. Add Superfoods for Extra Nutrients

Superfoods are called so for a reason – they are packed with essential nutrients and provide numerous health benefits. Add superfoods like berries, spinach, chia seeds, flaxseeds, and matcha powder to your smoothie to boost its nutritional content. These ingredients are also low in calories, making them a perfect addition to your weight loss smoothie.

7. Be Mindful of Portion Sizes

While smoothies can be a healthy addition to your weight loss diet, it is essential to pay attention to portion sizes. It is easy to overdo it with smoothies, especially if they taste delicious. Measure your ingredients and stick to recommended serving sizes to avoid consuming excess calories.

8. Keep a Balanced Diet

Incorporating smoothies into your weight loss diet does not mean you have to replace all your meals with them. It is crucial to maintain a balanced diet that includes a variety of whole foods like lean proteins, whole grains, and vegetables. Use smoothies as a supplement to your meals, and make sure to have a balance of all essential nutrients throughout the day.

9. Plan Ahead

Preparation is the key to success when it comes to weight loss. Planning your smoothie ingredients ahead of time can save you time and help you stick to your weight loss goals. You can freeze your ingredients, including fruits and vegetables, in individual portions to make smoothie-making more convenient.

10. Listen to Your Body

Lastly, it is essential to listen to your body and make adjustments as needed. Every individual's body is different, and what works for someone else may not work for you. Pay attention to how your body responds to different ingredients and make changes accordingly to find the perfect smoothie for your weight loss journey.

In conclusion, smoothies can be a powerful tool for weight loss when incorporated into a healthy and balanced diet. Through this book, we have explored various recipes that not only taste delicious but also provide essential nutrients and aid in weight loss. It is important to remember that while these smoothies can be beneficial in shedding pounds, they should not be relied on as the sole solution for weight loss. A healthy lifestyle, including regular exercise and mindful eating, should also be a part of the journey towards a slimmer and healthier self. With these delicious and nutritious smoothie recipes at your disposal, you are one step closer to achieving your weight loss goals. Cheers to a healthier and happier you!

www.ingramcontent.com/pod-product-compliance
Lightning Source LLC
Chambersburg PA
CBHW050836260726
48660CB00006B/2267